The Ultimate Medit Guide for E

Surprise Your Guests with These A
Appetizers Recipes

Lexi Robertson

Table of contents

Fennel Wild Rice

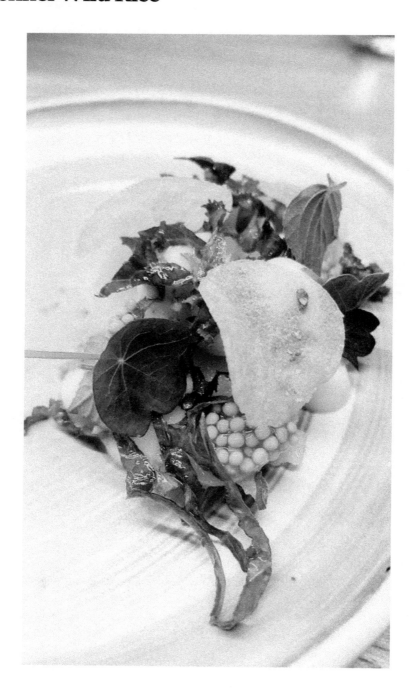

Difficulty Level: 2/5

Preparation time: 10 minutes

Cooking time: 11 minutes

Servings: 6

Ingredients:

1 tablespoon extra-virgin olive oil

1 cup diced fennel

½ red bell pepper, finely diced

½ cup chopped sweet onion

2 cups cooked wild rice

1 tablespoon chopped fresh parsley

Sea salt

Freshly ground black pepper

Directions:

In a large skillet over medium-high heat, heat the olive oil.

Add the fennel, red bell pepper, and onion. Sauté for about 6 minutes, or until tender.

Stir in the wild rice. Cook for about 5 minutes until heated through.

Add the parsley, and season with sea salt and pepper.

Nutrition:

Calories: 222;

Total Fat: 3g;

Saturated Fat: 0g;

Carbohydrates: 43g;

Fiber: 4g;

Protein: 8g

Brussels Sprouts with Pistachios
Difficulty Level: 2/5

Preparation time: 15 minutes

Cooking time: 15 minutes

Servings: 4

Ingredients:

1 pound Brussels sprouts, tough bottoms trimmed, halved lengthwise

4 shallots, peeled and quartered

1 tablespoon extra-virgin olive oil

Sea salt

Freshly ground black pepper

½ cup chopped roasted pistachios

Zest of ½ lemon

Juice of ½ lemon

Directions:

Preheat the oven to 400°F.

Line a baking sheet with aluminum foil and set aside.

In a large bowl, toss the Brussels sprouts and shallots with the olive oil until well coated.

Season with sea salt and pepper, and then spread the vegetables evenly on the sheet.

Bake for 15 minutes, or until tender and lightly caramelized.

Remove from the oven and transfer to a serving bowl.

Toss with the pistachios, lemon zest, and lemon juice. Serve warm.

Nutrition:

Calories: 126;

Total Fat: 7g;

Saturated Fat: 1g;

Carbohydrates: 14g;

Fiber: 5g;

Protein: 6g

Roasted Parmesan Broccoli
Difficulty Level: 2/5

Preparation time: 10 minutes

Cooking time: 10 minutes

Servings: 4

Ingredients:

2 heads broccoli, cut into small florets

2 tablespoons extra-virgin olive oil, plus more for greasing the baking sheet

2 teaspoons minced garlic

Zest of 1 lemon

Juice of 1 lemon

Pinch sea salt

½ cup grated Parmesan cheese

Directions:

Preheat the oven to 400°F.

Lightly grease a baking sheet with olive oil and set aside.

In a large bowl, toss the broccoli with the 2 tablespoons of olive oil, garlic, lemon zest, lemon juice, and sea salt

Spread the mixture on the baking sheet in a single layer and sprinkle with the Parmesan cheese.

Bake for about 10 minutes, or until tender. Transfer the broccoli to a serving dish and serve.

Nutrition:

Calories: 154;

Total Fat: 11g;

Saturated Fat: 3g;

Carbohydrates: 10g;

Fiber: 4;

Protein: 9g

Mashed Celeriac

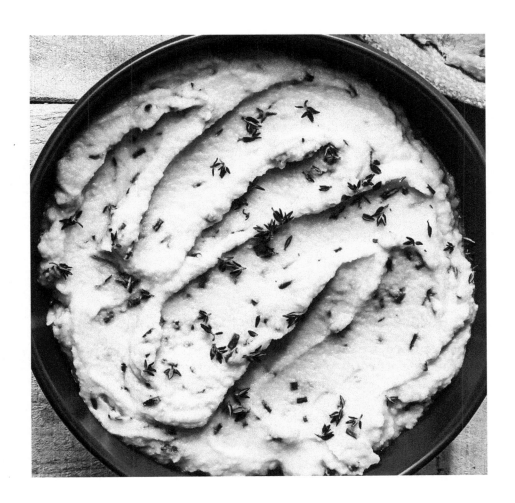

Difficulty Level: 2/5

Preparation time: 10 minutes

Cooking time: 20 minutes

Servings: 4

Ingredients:

2 celeriac (celery root), washed, peeled, and diced

2 teaspoons extra-virgin olive oil

1 tablespoon honey

½ teaspoon ground nutmeg

Sea salt

Freshly ground black pepper

Directions:

Preheat the oven to 400°F.

Line a baking sheet with aluminum foil and set aside.

In a large bowl, toss together the celeriac and olive oil. Spread the celeriac pieces evenly on the baking sheet, and roast for about 20 minutes until very tender and lightly caramelized. Transfer to a large bowl.

Add the honey and nutmeg. Use a potato masher to mash the ingredients until fluffy.

Season with sea salt and pepper before serving.

Nutrition:

Calories: 136;

Total Fat: 3g;

Saturated Fat: 1g;

Carbohydrates: 26g;

Fiber: 4g;

Protein: 4g

Herbed Yogurt Dip
Difficulty Level: 1/5

Preparation time: 10 minutes

Cooking time: 0 minutes

Servings: 4

Ingredients:

1 cup plain Greek yogurt

Zest of ½ lemon

Juice of ½ lemon

1 tablespoon finely chopped fresh chives

2 teaspoons chopped fresh dill

2 teaspoons chopped fresh thyme

1 teaspoon chopped fresh parsley

½ teaspoon minced garlic

Pinch sea salt

Directions:

In a medium bowl, stir together the yogurt, lemon zest, lemon juice, chives, dill, thyme, parsley, and garlic until very well blended.

Season with the sea salt and transfer to a sealed container.

Keep refrigerated for up to 2 weeks.

Nutrition:

Calories: 59;

Total Fat: 4g;

Saturated Fat: 2g;

Carbohydrates: 5g;

Fiber: 4g;

Protein: 2g

Southwest Pizza
Difficulty Level: 2/5

Preparation time: 15 minutes

Cooking time: 10 minutes

Servings: 4

Ingredients:

4 (6-inch) whole-wheat pita breads

1 tablespoon extra-virgin olive oil

2 cups canned sodium-free white navy beans, drained and rinsed

1 scallion, white and green parts, finely chopped

1 jalapeño pepper, seeded and finely chopped

1 teaspoon ground cumin

1 tomato, diced

1 yellow bell pepper, thinly sliced

½ cup crumbled feta cheese

4 teaspoons chopped fresh cilantro

Directions:

Preheat the oven to 400°F.

Place the pita breads on a baking sheet and lightly brush both sides with olive oil. Bake for about 5 minutes until golden brown and crispy, turning once.

In a medium bowl, mash together the beans, scallion, jalapeño, and cumin to form a chunky paste.

Evenly divide the bean mixture among the toasted pita breads, spreading it to the edges.

Top each with tomato, yellow bell pepper, and feta cheese.

Bake the pizzas for about 3 minutes until the cheese is slightly melted.

Sprinkle with cilantro and serve.

Nutrition:

Calories: 387;

Total Fat: 9g;

Saturated Fat: 3g;

Carbohydrates: 64g;

Fiber: 16g;

Protein: 17g

Spinach Chicken Pizza
Difficulty Level: 2/5

Preparation time: 15 minutes

Cooking time: 15 minutes

Servings: 4

Ingredients:

1 (9-inch) pizza crust, homemade or premade

½ teaspoon extra-virgin olive oil

1 cup chopped tomato

¼ teaspoon red pepper flakes

2 cups chopped blanched fresh spinach

1 tablespoon chopped fresh basil

1 cup chopped cooked chicken breast

1 cup shredded Asiago cheese

Directions:

Preheat the oven to 400°F.

Prepare the pizza dough according to your recipe or package instructions and roll it out to form a 9-inch crust. Transfer the crust to a baking sheet, and brush the edges lightly with olive oil.

Spread the tomato and red pepper flakes over the pizza leaving the oiled crust bare.

Arrange the spinach and basil over the tomato, and scatter the chopped chicken on the spinach. Top with the Asiago cheese.

Bake the pizza for about 15 minutes until the crust is crispy and the cheese is melted.

Nutrition:

Calories: 255;

Total Fat: 11g;

Saturated Fat: 5g;

Carbohydrates: 17g;

Fiber: 2g;

Protein: 23g

Linguine with Cherry Tomatoes

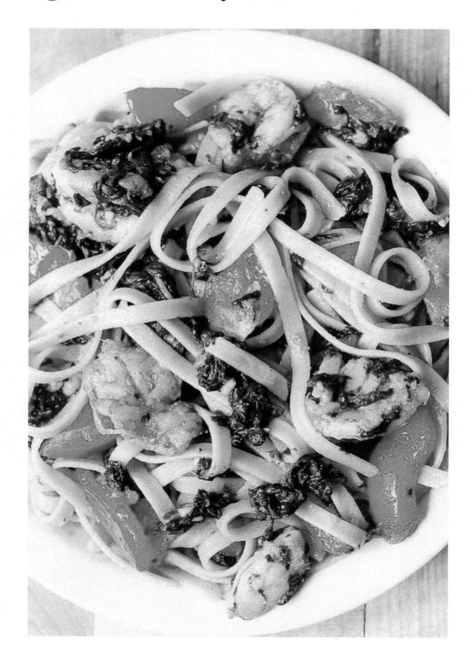

Difficulty Level: 2/5

Preparation time: 10 minutes

Cooking time: 15 minutes

Servings: 4

Ingredients:

2 pounds cherry tomatoes

3 tablespoons extra-virgin olive oil

2 tablespoons balsamic vinegar

2 teaspoons minced garlic

Pinch freshly ground black pepper

¾ pound whole-wheat linguine pasta

1 tablespoon chopped fresh oregano

¼ cup crumbled feta cheese

Directions:

Preheat the oven to 350°F.

Line a baking sheet with parchment paper and set aside.

In a large bowl, toss the cherry tomatoes with 2 tablespoons of olive oil, the balsamic vinegar, garlic, and pepper until well coated. Spread the tomatoes evenly on the prepared sheet and roast for about 15 minutes until they are softened and burst open.

While the tomatoes roast, cook the pasta according to package directions. Drain and transfer to a large bowl.

Toss the pasta with the remaining 1 tablespoon of olive oil.

Add the roasted tomatoes, taking care to get all the juices and bits from the baking sheet. Toss to combine.

To serve, top with the oregano and feta cheese.

Nutrition:

Calories: 397;

Total Fat: 15g;

Saturated Fat: 3g;

Carbohydrates: 55g;

Fiber: 6g;

Protein: 13g

Linguine with Tomato Clam Sauce
Difficulty Level: 2/5

Preparation time: 10 minutes

Cooking time: 10minutes

Servings: 4

Ingredients:

1 pound linguine

Pinch sea salt

1 teaspoon extra-virgin olive oil

1 tablespoon minced garlic

1 teaspoon chopped fresh thyme

½ teaspoon red pepper flakes

1 (15-ounce) can sodium-free diced tomatoes, drained

1 (15-ounce) can whole baby clams, with their juice

Sea salt

Freshly ground black pepper

2 tablespoons chopped fresh parsley

Directions:

Cook the linguine according to the package directions.

While the linguine cooks, heat the olive oil in a large skillet over medium heat.

the garlic, thyme, and red pepper flakes. Sauté for about 3 minutes until softened.

Stir in the tomatoes and clams. Bring the sauce to a boil, reduce the heat to low, and simmer for 5 minutes.

Season with sea salt and pepper.

Drain the cooked pasta and toss it with the sauce.

Garnish with the parsley and serve.

Nutrition:

Calories: 394;

Total Fat: 5g;

Saturated Fat: 0g;

Carbohydrates: 66g;

Fiber: 7g;

Protein: 23g

Angel Hair with Asparagus-Kale Pesto
Difficulty Level: 2/5

Preparation time: 10 minutes

Cooking time: 10 minutes

Servings: 6

Ingredients:

¾ pound asparagus, woody ends removed, and coarsely chopped

¼ pound kale, thoroughly washed

½ cup grated Asiago cheese

¼ cup fresh basil

¼ cup extra-virgin olive oil

Juice of 1 lemon

Sea salt

Freshly ground black pepper

1 pound angel hair pasta

Zest of 1 lemon

Directions:

In a food processor, pulse the asparagus and kale until very finely chopped.

Add the Asiago cheese, basil, olive oil, and lemon juice and pulse to form a smooth pesto.

Season with sea salt and pepper and set aside.

Cook the pasta al dente according to the package directions. Drain and transfer to a large bowl.

Add the pesto, tossing well to coat.

Sprinkle with lemon zest and serve.

Nutrition:

Calories: 283;

Total Fat: 12g;

Saturated Fat: 2g;

Carbohydrates: 33g;

Fiber: 2g;

Protein: 10g

Cucumber Hummus Sandwiches
Difficulty Level: 1/5

Preparation time: 5 minutes

Cooking time: 0 minutes

Servings: 1

Ingredients:

10 round slices cucumber

5 teaspoons hummus

Instructions:

Add 1 teaspoon hummus on one slice of cucumber. Top with another slice and serve.

Nutritional info (per serving):

54 calories;

2.1 g fat;

7 g total carbs;

2 g protein

Blackberries Caprese Skewers
Difficulty Level: 2/5

Preparation time: 15 minutes

Cooking time: 0 minutes

Servings: 4

Ingredients:

½ cup cherry tomatoes

4 fresh basil leaves

4 blackberries

¼ cup baby mozzarella balls

Directions:

Put blackberries, tomatoes, mozzarella balls, and basil on skewers.

Once done, serve.

Nutritional info (per serving):

40 calories;

1.7 g fat;

4 g total carbs;

2 g protein

Tomato-Basil Skewers
Difficulty Level: 1/5

Preparation time: 15 minutes

Cooking time: 0 minutes

Servings: 6

Ingredients:

16 cherry tomatoes

16 fresh basil leaves

16 small fresh mozzarella balls

olive oil

salt and black pepper

Instructions:

Put mozzarella, basil, and tomatoes on skewers.

Add the oil and season well.

Once done, serve.

Nutritional info (per serving):

46 calories;

3.3 g fat;

1 g total carbs;

2.8 g protein

Fig and Ricotta Toast
Difficulty Level: 2/5

Preparation time: 10 minutes

Cooking time: 0 minutes

Servings: 1

Ingredients:

1 fresh fig dried, sliced

1 slice crusty whole-grain bread

¼ cup part-skim ricotta cheese

1 teaspoon honey

1 teaspoon sliced almonds, toasted

pinch flaky sea salt

Directions:

Toast the bread and add the figs, ricotta cheese, and almonds on it.

Add honey on top, season with sea salt, and serve.

Nutritional info (per serving):

252 calories;

9.1 g fat;

32.1 g total carbs;

12.5 g protein

Date Wraps
Difficulty Level: 1/5

Preparation time: 10 minutes

Cooking time: 0 minutes

Servings: 16 bites

Ingredients:

16 whole pitted dates

16 thin slices prosciutto

pepper

Directions:

Place prosciutto slice flat on a plate. Put a date into it and wrap the slice around it.

Repeat with the remaining, season with pepper and serve.

Nutritional info (per serving):

35 calories;

0.8 g fat;

5.6 g total carbs;

2.2 g protein

Easy Stuffed Peppers
Difficulty Level: 2/5

Preparation time: 5 minutes

Cooking time: 10 minutes

Servings: 4

Ingredients:

2 tablespoon pesto sauce

4 red peppers

1 lb. cooked tomato rice

2 cups goat cheese, sliced

handful black olives, pitted

Directions:

Cut the top of the red peppers and scoop out the seeds. Place the peppers on the plate, cut side up, and microwave for 6 minutes on high.

Mix the rice with pesto with a handful of black olives, and 1 3/8 cup cheese. Add this mixture on the peppers and top with the remaining cheese. Cook for 10 minutes.

Serve.

Nutritional info (per serving):

387 calories;

17 g fat;

46 g total carbs;

15 g protein

Buttery Carrot Sticks
Difficulty Level: 2/5

Preparation time: 10 minutes

Cooking time: 15 minutes

Serves: 4

Ingredients:

1 pound carrot, cut into sticks

4 garlic cloves, minced

¼ cup chicken stock

1 teaspoon rosemary, chopped

A pinch of salt and black pepper

2 tablespoons olive oil

2 tablespoons ghee, melted

Directions:

Set the Pressure Pot on Sauté mode, add the oil and the ghee, heat them up, add the garlic and brown for 1 minute.

Add the rest of the ingredients, put the lid on and cook on High for 14 minutes.

Release the pressure naturally for 10 minutes, arrange the carrot sticks on a platter and serve.

Nutrition:

Calories 142,

Fat 4g,

Fiber 2g,

Carbohydrates 5g,

Protein 7g

Cajun Walnuts and Olives Bowls
Difficulty Level: 2/5

Preparation time: 10 minutes

Cooking time: 10 minutes

Serves: 2

Ingredients:

½ pound walnuts, chopped

A pinch of salt and black pepper

1 and ½ cups black olives, pitted

½ tablespoon Cajun seasoning

2 garlic cloves, minced

1 red chili pepper, chopped

¼ cup veggie stock

2 tablespoon tomato puree

Directions:

In your Pressure Pot, combine the walnuts with the olives and the rest of the ingredients, put the lid on and cook on High 10 minutes.

Release the pressure fast for 5 minutes, divide the mix into small bowls and serve as an appetizer.

Nutrition:

Calories 105,

Fat 1g,

Fiber 1g,

Carbohydrates 4g,

Protein 7g

Mango Salsa

Difficulty Level: 2/5

Preparation time: 10 minutes

Cooking time: 10 minutes

Serves: 2

Ingredients:

2 mangoes, peeled and cubed

½ tablespoon sweet paprika

2 garlic cloves, minced

2 tablespoons cilantro, chopped

1 tablespoon spring onions, chopped

1 cup cherry tomatoes, cubed

1 cup avocado, peeled, pitted and cubed

A pinch of salt and black pepper

1 tablespoon olive oil

¼ cup tomato puree

½ cup kalamata olives, pitted and sliced

Directions:

In your Pressure Pot, combine the mangoes with the paprika and the rest of the ingredients except the cilantro, put the lid on and cook on High for 5 minutes.

Release the pressure fast for 5 minutes, divide the mix into small bowls, sprinkle the cilantro on top and serve.

Nutrition:

Calories 123,

Fat 4g,

Fiber 1g,
Carbs 3g,
Protein 5g

Crisp Spiced Cauliflower with Feta Cheese
Difficulty Level: 2/5

Preparation time: 5 minutes

Cooking time: 10 minutes

Serves: 4

Ingredients:

3/4 lb cauliflower, chopped

1/2 Tbsp. ground toasted cumin seeds

1 garlic clove, grated

2 Tbsp. crumbled feta cheese

1 1/2 Tbsp. freshly squeezed lemon juice

1 Tbsp. chopped fresh flat leaf parsley

Chili flakes

Sweet smoked paprika

Sea salt

Canola oil

Directions:

Place a skillet over high flame and heat just enough canola oil to cover the bottom.

Allow the oil to smoke slightly, then add the chopped cauliflower and stir fry for about 2 minutes or until browned and crisp. Season with salt.

Reduce to medium flame as you continue to stir fry the cauliflower. Sprinkle in the cumin, lemon juice, grated garlic, and a dash of chili flakes, then stir well to combine.

Transfer the cauliflower to a platter, then top with feta, parsley, and a dash of paprika. Serve right away.

Nutrition:

Calories 300,

Fat 19.3 g,

Carbohydrates 30.6 g,

Sugar 8.8 g,

Protein 3.4 g,

Cholesterol 0 mg

Spring Peas and Beans with Zesty Thyme Yogurt Sauce
Difficulty Level: 3/5

Preparation time: 5 minutes

Cooking time: 10 minutes

Serves: 4

Ingredients:

3/4 lb fresh shelling beans, shelled

3/4 lb fresh peas (such as English peas, edamame, etc.), shelled

1 lb pole beans, preferably assorted (such as purple wax, Romano, and yellow)

6 young pea shoots

1/2 tsp. ground sumac

1 1/2 Tbsp. extra virgin olive oil

Sea salt

For the Zesty Thyme Yogurt Sauce:

1/4 cup Greek yogurt

1 1/2 Tbsp. fresh thyme leaves

1 garlic clove, grated

1/2 lemon, juiced and zested

Cayenne

Sea salt

Directions:

Combine all the ingredients for the yogurt sauce in a bowl, then season to taste with salt and cayenne. Cover the bowl and refrigerate until ready to serve.

Prepare a bowl of ice water and set aside.

Boil some salted water in a saucepan, then add the fresh beans and peas. Boil for 2 minutes, or until tender, then remove immediately with a metal mesh strainer and plunge into the ice water to prevent them from being soggy.

Blot the peas and beans dry using paper towels, then place in a large bowl and set aside.

Refill the bowl of ice water.

Boil the salted water in the saucepan again, then add the pole beans and cook for 2 minutes or until almost tender. Remove immediately with a metal mesh strainer and plunge into the ice water to prevent them from being soggy.

Blot the pole beans dry using paper towels, then add to the bowl of peas and beans. Toss everything to combine.

Drizzle the olive oil over the peas and beans, then season with salt and sumac. Toss well to combine, then add the yogurt sauce on top. Garnish with pea shoots and thyme, then serve right away.

Nutrition:

Calories 153,

Fat 0.5 g,

Carbohydrates 39.1 g,

Sugar 25.7 g,

Protein 1.2 g,

Cholesterol 0 mg

Breakfast Pita

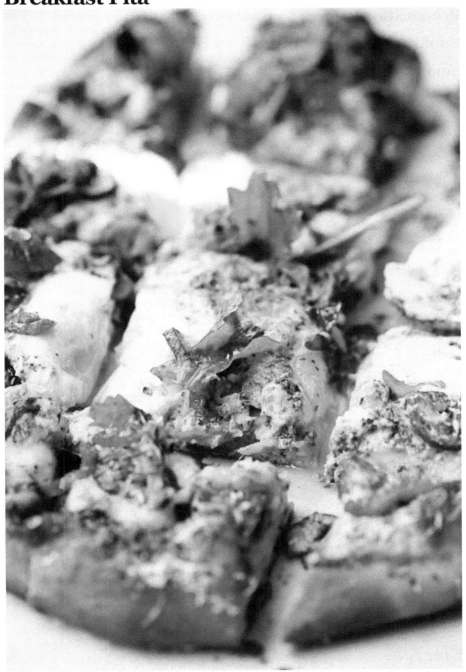

Difficulty Level: 2/5

Preparation Time: 15 minutes

Cooking time: 15 minutes

Servings: 4

Ingredients:

4 pita breads

2 eggs, whisked

4 oz. ham, chopped

1 tablespoon olive oil

¼ teaspoon salt

4 oz. Parmesan, grated

1 cup water

Directions:

Rub the pitas with the olive oil. Place them in ramekins and put them on the trivet.

Combine the whisked eggs, ham, salt, and grated cheese in the mixing bowl.

Pour the egg mixture into the ramekins with pita and transfer the trivet into the Pressure Pot.

Pour the water into the bottom of the Pressure Pot bowl.

Close the lid and cook the pitas for 15 minutes on High pressure.

Do a natural pressure release and serve the breakfast!

Nutrition:

Calories 199,

Fat 15.1,

Fiber 2,

Carbohydrates 45.4,

Protein 22.6

Beef with Pesto Sandwich

Difficulty Level: 2/5

Preparation time: 5 minutes

Cooking Time: 20 minutes

Servings: 4

Ingredients:

4 slices mozzarella cheese

½ lb. thinly sliced roast beef deli

¼ cup basil pesto

2 tbsp softened butter

8 slices, ½-inch thick Italian bread

Directions:

Spread the butter on one side of four of the bread slices, then top with pesto and evenly spread.

Top with beef, then cheese slices and cover with the un-buttered bread slice.

Place on a Panini pan and grill until crispy. Serve and enjoy.

Nutrition:

Calories per Serving: 248;

Carbohydrates: 2.5g;

Protein: 23.3g;

Fat: 15.8g

Classic Steak Panini
Difficulty Level: 2/5

Preparation time: 5 minutes

Cooking time: 12 minutes

Servings: 2

Ingredients:

2 tbsp yellow mustard

2 tbsp softened butter

1 baguette or ciabatta roll

Ground pepper and salt

2 thin slices of minute steaks

2 large onions peeled and sliced

2 tbsp olive oil

Directions:

On a heated skillet pour half of the oil and cook onions until browned and translucent, around ten minutes.

Season steak with salt and pepper. Then, gather thee onions on one end of the skillet and pour in the remaining oil as you pan fry the seasoned steak on high heat.

Cooking each side for at least 45 seconds and remove from fire and set aside.

Halve your bread lengthwise and arrange the steaks topped by onions and cover with the other bread half. Grill your sandwich in a Panini pan for at least 3 minutes.

Serve with your favorite condiment.

Nutrition:

Calories per Serving: 529;

Carbohydrates: 27.7g;

Protein: 14.0g;

Fat: 41.8g

Grilled Sandwich with Goat Cheese

Difficulty Level: 2/5

Preparation time: 10 minutes

Cooking time: 8 minutes

Servings: 4

Ingredients:

½ cup soft goat cheese

4 Kaiser rolls 2-oz

¼ tsp freshly ground black pepper

¼ tsp salt

1/3 cup chopped basil

Cooking spray

4 big Portobello mushroom caps

1 yellow bell pepper, cut in half and seeded

1 red bell pepper, cut in half and seeded

1 garlic clove, minced

1 tbsp olive oil

¼ cup balsamic vinegar

Directions:

In a large bowl, mix garlic, olive oil and balsamic vinegar. Add mushroom and bell peppers. Gently mix to coat. Remove veggies from vinegar and discard vinegar mixture.

Coat with cooking spray a grill rack and the grill preheated to medium high fire.

Place mushrooms and bell peppers on the grill and grill for 4 minutes per side. Remove from grill and let cool a bit.

Into thin strips, cut the bell peppers.

In a small bowl, combine black pepper, salt, basil and sliced bell peppers.

Horizontally, cut the Kaiser rolls and evenly spread cheese on the cut side.

Arrange 1 Portobello per roll, top with 1/3 bell pepper mixture and cover with the other half of the roll.

Grill the rolls as you press down on them to create a Panini like line on the bread. Grill until bread is toasted.

Nutrition:

Calories per Serving: 317;

Carbohydrates: 41.7g;

Protein: 14.0g;

Fat: 10.5g

Fried Green Tomatoes
Difficulty Level: 2/5

Preparation time: 10 minutes

Cooking time: 8 minutes

Servings: 4

Ingredients

1 tablespoon Vegetable Oil

½ teaspoon Black Pepper

½ teaspoon Salt

½ cup Bread Crumbs

½ cup Cornmeal

1 cup All-purpose Flour

½ cup Milk

2 Eggs

4 Green Tomatoes

Directions

Pour the vegetable oil into a large pan and begin to heat it up into a medium heat.

While the oil heats, you will want to prepare your tomatoes by slicing them into half inch thick pieces.

Be sure to throw the ends out as you will have no need for them. In a bowl, mix together the milk and the eggs.

Place your flour onto a plate and line up with the bowl that is holding the milk and eggs.

On a third plate, mix together your breadcrumbs, cornmeal, pepper, and salt.

Now that these are prepared, dip your tomato pieces in the liquid mixture, the flour, and then the breadcrumb mixture. Be sure to coat the tomatoes before tossing them into the vegetable oil.

Fry the tomatoes for five minutes on either side or until golden brown. Portion them out and enjoy as a side dish or a nice, healthy snack!

Nutrition:

Calories per Serving: 298;

Carbs: 61.1g;

Protein: 7.4g;

Fat: 5.0g

One-of-a-Kind Veggie Slaw
Difficulty Level: 2/5

Preparation time: 10 minutes

Cooking time: 20 minutes

Servings: 6

Ingredients:

2 tsp salt

2 tbsp Bavarian seasoning

½ cup lightly packed fresh mint leaves

½ cup fresh lemon juice

½ cup roasted and shelled pistachios, roughly chopped

6 oz dried cranberries

4 bacon strips, cooked to a crisp (keep rendered fat) and chopped to bits

1/3 cup extra virgin olive oil (use rendered fat from bacon to reach ½ cup)

2 lbs. Brussels sprouts, cleaned and trimmed of large stem pieces

Directions:

Shred Brussels sprouts in a food processor. Transfer into a large salad bowl.

In a small bowl mix salt, Bavarian seasoning, mint and lemon juice.

Then slowly add oil while whisking continuously and vigorously. Add more seasoning to taste if needed.

Pour half of dressing into the salad bowl, toss to mix and add more if needed.

Top salad with bacon pieces, dried cranberries and pistachios before serving.

Nutrition:

Calories per Serving: 343.8;

Carbohydrates: 38.7g;

Protein: 9.7g;

Fat: 20.0g

Ratatouille Grilled Style
Difficulty Level: 2/5

Preparation time:

Cooking time: 20 minutes

Servings: 4

Ingredients:

2 tbsp walnuts, toasted and chopped

2 tbsp apple cider

2 tbsp extra virgin olive oil

2 medium yellow squash, cut into ¼" rounds

1 large zucchini, cut into ¼" rounds

1 large zucchini, cut into ¼" rounds

1 large Portobello mushroom cap, cut into ¼" slices

1 medium eggplant, cut into ¼" rounds

1 red bell pepper, quartered, stems and seeds removed

1 large red onion, cut into ¼" slices

Directions:

Preheat grill to medium high and lightly grease grill pan with cooking spray.

Place all sliced veggies in grill pan and drizzle with olive oil. Toss well to coat.

Place in grill and grill for ten minutes. Toss vegetables to ensure even heating and continue grilling for another 10 minutes.

Toss vegetables and check if lightly charred and cooked through. If needed, grill some more to desired doneness.

Transfer grilled veggies into salad bowl, add walnuts and zero belly dressing. T

Toss to combine well, serve and enjoy.

Nutrition:

Calories per Serving: 212;

Carbs: 27.6g;

Protein: 7.4g;

Fat: 10.6g

Cooked Beef Mushroom Egg
Difficulty Level: 2/5

Preparation time: 10 minutes

Cooking time: 15 minutes

Servings: 2

Ingredients:

¼ cup cooked beef, diced

6 eggs

4 mushrooms, diced

Salt and pepper to taste

12 ounces spinach

2 onions, chopped

A dash of onion powder

¼ green bell pepper, chopped

A dash of garlic powder

Directions:

In a skillet, toss the beef for 3 minutes or until crispy.

Take off the heat and add to a plate.

Add the onion, bell pepper, and mushroom in the skillet.

Add the rest of the ingredients.

Toss for about 4 minutes.

Return the beef to the skillet and toss for another minute.

Serve hot.

Nutrition:

Calories per serving: 213;

Protein: 14.5g;

Carbs: 3.4g;

Fat: 15.7g

Eggs over Kale Hash
Difficulty Level: 2/5

Preparation time: 10 minutes

Cooking time: 20 minutes

Servings: 4

Ingredients:

4 large eggs

1 bunch chopped kale

Dash of ground nutmeg

2 sweet potatoes, cubed

1 14.5-ounce can of chicken broth

Directions:

In a large non-stick skillet, bring the chicken broth to a simmer. Add the sweet potatoes and season slightly with salt and pepper.

Add a dash of nutmeg to improve the flavor.

Cook until the sweet potatoes become soft, around 10 minutes. Add kale and season with salt and pepper. Continue cooking for four minutes or until kale has wilted. Set aside.

Using the same skillet, heat 1 tablespoon of olive oil over medium high heat.

Cook the eggs sunny side up until the whites become opaque and the yolks have set. Top the kale hash with the eggs. Serve immediately.

Nutrition:

Calories per serving: 158;

Protein: 9.8g;

Carbohydrates 18.5g;

Fat: 5.6g

Italian Scrambled Eggs

Difficulty Level: 2/5

Preparation time: 5 minutes

Cooking Time: 7 minutes

Servings: 1

Ingredients:

1 teaspoon balsamic vinegar

2 large eggs

¼ teaspoon rosemary, minced

½ cup cherry tomatoes

1 ½ cup kale, chopped

½ teaspoon olive oil

Directions:

Melt the olive oil in a skillet over medium high heat.

Sauté the kale and add rosemary and salt to taste. Add three tablespoons of water to prevent the kale from burning at the bottom of the pan. Cook for three to four minutes.

Add the tomatoes and stir.

Push the vegetables on one side of the skillet and add the eggs. Season with salt and pepper to taste.

Scramble the eggs then fold in the tomatoes and kales.

Nutrition:

Calories per serving: 230;

Protein: 16.4g;

Carbs: 15.0g;

Fat: 12.4g

Scrambled Eggs with Feta 'n Mushrooms
Difficulty Level: 2/5

Preparation time: 5 minutes

Cooking time: 6 minutes

Servings: 1

Ingredients:

Pepper to taste

2 tbsp feta cheese

1 whole egg

2 egg whites

1 cup fresh spinach, chopped

½ cup fresh mushrooms, sliced

Cooking spray

Directions:

On medium high fire, place a nonstick fry pan and grease with cooking spray.

Once hot, add spinach and mushrooms.

Sauté until spinach is wilted, around 2-3 minutes.

Meanwhile, in a bowl whisk well egg, egg whites, and cheese. Season with pepper.

Pour egg mixture into pan and scramble until eggs are cooked through, around 3-4 minutes.

Serve and enjoy with a piece of toast or brown rice.

Nutrition:

Calories per serving: 211;

Protein: 18.6g;

Carbs: 7.4g;

Fat: 11.9g

Black Bean Hummus

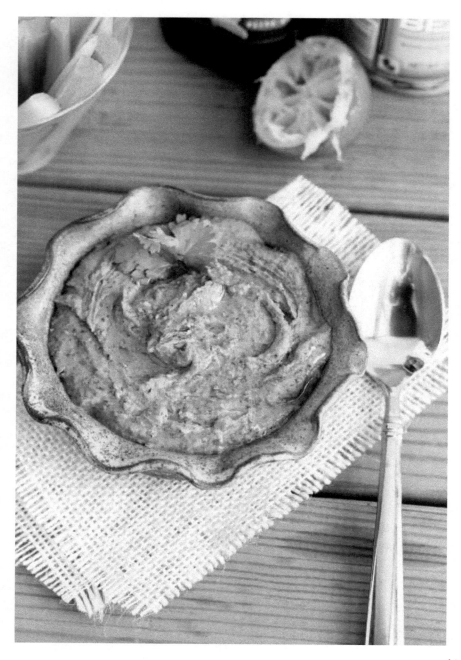

Difficulty Level: 2/5

Preparation time: 5 min

Cooking time: -min

Servings: 2

Ingredients:

2 (15.5 ounce) cans black beans

2 cups low-fat cottage cheese

3 tablespoons almond butter

1 garlic clove, sliced

2 tablespoons extra-virgin olive oil

3 tablespoons red wine vinegar

3/4 teaspoon sea salt

1/2 teaspoon ground cumin

1 teaspoon ground coriander

1/4 cup fresh parsley

2 tablespoons orange zest

Freshly ground black pepper to taste

10-12 stalks of celery, cut into thirds

Directions:

Mix all the ingredients in a food processor, except celery, and puree till smooth. If necessary, scrap down the sides.

Move to a bowl and serve with celery. *Enjoy!*

Nutrition: (Per serving)

Calories:218kcal;

Fat:7.5g;

Saturated fat:1.5g;

Cholesterol:10mg;

Carbohydrate:20g;

Sugar:4.5g;

Fiber:5.5g;

Protein:16g

Portobello Mushroom Delight
Difficulty Level: 2/5

Preparation time: 5 min

Cooking time: 15 min

Servings: 2

Ingredients:

2 Portobello mushroom caps (around 3 ounces each)

2 tablespoons soft goat cheese

2 tablespoons sundried tomatoes

2 large eggs

extra-virgin (organic) olive oil spray

Salt and pepper to taste

Basil for garnish

Directions:

Preheat the oven to 400 degrees Fahrenheit.

From the mushroom caps remove the stems and with a spoon scrape out the gills.

Use cooking spray to spray both sides of the mushroom and set them onto the baking sheet.

Place into each mushroom 1 tablespoon of goat cheese, where the gills used to be.

Finely chop sun-dried tomatoes and sprinkle into each mushroom cap 1 tablespoon of them.

Into each mushroom cap crack an egg, striving to get the yolk to sit in the cavity where the steam was, so it doesn't move around.

Transfer the baking sheet to the oven and bake for 15 minutes.

Once the eggs are done to your liking, transfer them from the oven and season with salt and pepper.

Top with sliced basil and serve. *Enjoy!*

Tip: Make this into a meal by tossing arugula, baby kale, or other lettuce greens in lemon juice, olive oil, salt and pepper and having as a side salad.

Nutrition: (Per serving)

Calories:122kcal;

Fat:8.5g;

Saturated fat:3g;

Cholesterol:223mg;

Carbohydrate:2g;

Sugar:1g;

Fiber:0.5g;

Protein:8.5g

Tuna Salad On Crackers
Difficulty Level: 1/5

Preparation time: 10 min

Cooking time: - min

Servings: 4

Ingredients:

1 (7 ounce) can Albacore Tuna in brine water

2 tablespoons celery, finely chopped

3 tablespoons Canola Oil Mayonnaise

1/2 teaspoon lemon pepper

11/2 tablespoons red onion, finely chopped

1/4 teaspoon dried dill weed

16 Ritz Crackers

2 green leaf lettuce leaves, torn

Fresh dill, for garnish (optional)

Directions:

In a mixing bowl place tuna and mash up to desired size pieces. Add in celery, mayonnaise, lemon pepper, onion, and dill weed. Mix well to combine.

On top of each cracker place a piece of torn lettuce and top that with 1 tablespoon of tuna salad. Decorate with a piece of fresh dill weed, if desired and serve. *Enjoy!*

Nutrition (4 crackers)

Calories:165kcal;

Fat:7g;

Saturated fat:1g;

Cholesterol:19mg;

Carbohydrate:9g;

Sugar:1g;

Fiber:1g;

Protein:13g

Fresh Fruit Crumble Muesli

Difficulty Level: 1/5

Preparation Time: *20 minutes*

Cooking Time: *0 minutes*

Servings: *4*

Ingredients:

1 cup gluten-free rolled oats

¼ cup chopped pecans

¼ cup almonds

4 pitted Medjool dates

1 teaspoon vanilla extract

¼ teaspoon ground cinnamon

1 cup sliced fresh strawberries

1 nectarine, pitted and chopped

2 kiwis, peeled and chopped

½ cup blueberries

1 cup low-fat plain Greek yogurt

Directions:

In a food processor, combine the oats, pecans, almonds, dates, vanilla, and cinnamon and pulse until the mixture resembles coarse crumbs.

In a medium bowl, stir together the strawberries, nectarine, kiwis, and blueberries until well mixed. Divide the fruit and yogurt between bowls and top each bowl with the oat mixture. Serve.

Nutrition:

Calories: 258

Total fat: 6g

Saturated fat: 0g

Carbohydrates: 45g

Sugar: 28g

Fiber: 7g

Protein: 11g

Crispy Squid with Capers

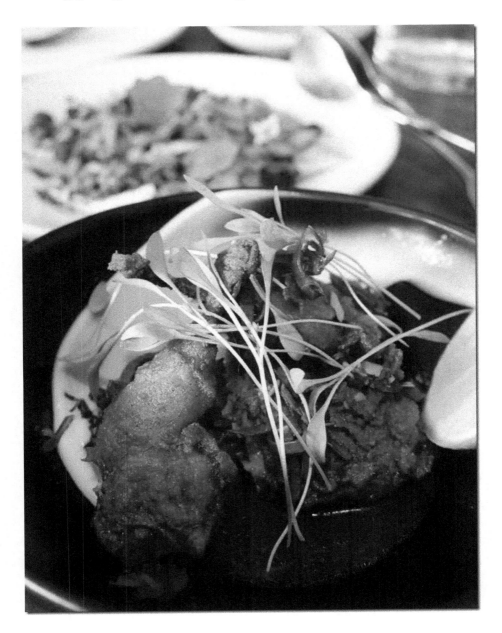

Difficulty Level: 2/5

Preparation Time: 5 minutes

Cooking time: 20 minutes

Servings: 3

Ingredients:

1 garlic clove, crushed

2½ tablespoons mayonnaise

Olive oil, for frying

3.5 oz. whole wheat flour

5 oz. baby squid, cleaned and sliced into thick rings

1 tablespoon caper, drained and finely chopped

Lemon wedges, to serve

Directions:

Combine together squid, capers and whole wheat flour in a bowl.

Heat oil in a skillet and deep fry capers and squids until golden.

Dish out the capers and squid in a plate.

Serve with mayonnaise, garlic and lemon wedges.

Nutrition:

Calories 213

Total Fat 5.1 g

Saturated Fat 0.8 g

Cholesterol 113 mg

Total Carbs 29.9 g

Dietary Fiber 1 g

Sugar 0.9 g

Protein 11 g

Garlic Bread Pizzas
Difficulty Level: 2/5

Preparation Time: 10 minutes

Cooking time: 15 minutes

Servings: 8

Ingredients:

For the dough

2 pounds strong whole wheat flour, plus extra for rolling

4 tablespoons olive oil

2 sachets fast-action yeast

2 teaspoons salt

For the topping

½ cup almond butter, softened

2 teaspoons balsamic vinegar

2 tablespoons extra-virgin olive oil

4 garlic cloves, crushed

3 cups mozzarella, drained

½ cup basil leaves, roughly chopped

8 tomatoes, roughly chopped

Directions:

Preheat the oven to 330 degrees F and grease 4 baking sheets.

Knead together all the ingredients for the dough in a bowl and roll out into 16 equal pieces.

Mix together garlic and butter in a bowl and pour over the dough.

Organize these pieces into the baking sheets and top with mozzarella cheese.

Transfer into the oven and bake for about 15 minutes.

Top with rest of the ingredients and immediately serve.

Nutrition:

Calories 629

Total Fat 21.8 g

Saturated Fat 9.6 g

Cholesterol 36 mg

Total Carbs 92.2 g

Dietary Fiber 4.6 g

Sugar 3.6 g

Protein 16 g

Falafel

Difficulty Level: 2/5

Preparation Time: 15 minutes

Cooking time: 4 minutes

Servings: 6

Ingredients:

1 cup chickpeas, cooked

1 onion, finely chopped

2 tablespoons flour

1 tablespoon chopped parsley

1 teaspoon ground coriander

2 tablespoons olive oil

1 teaspoon salt

Directions:

Blend the cooked chickpeas, chopped onion, and parsley.

When the mixture is smooth, add the flour and ground coriander.

Blend the mixture for 20 seconds more.

Transfer the mixture to bowl.

Make small balls from the chickpea mixture and press them gently into a flat disc.

Pour the olive oil into the Pressure Pot bowl.

Add the falafel and use the saute mode to cook the falafel for 2 minutes on each side.

Cool the cooked falafel slightly and serve!

Nutrition:

Calories 178,

Fat 6.7,

Fiber 6.3,

Carbs 23.9,

Protein 6.9

Chicken Sandwich
Difficulty Level: 2/5

Preparation Time: 10 minutes

Cooking time: 15 minutes

Servings: 4

Ingredients:

7 oz. chicken fillets

1 tablespoon olive oil

1 teaspoon salts

½ teaspoon ground black pepper

4 oz. French bread, sliced

1 tomato, sliced

1 cup water

2 oz. lettuce

Directions:

Cut the chicken fillet into strips.

Sprinkle the chicken with the salt and ground black pepper.

Add the olive oil and stir the meat well.

Pour the water into the Pressure Pot.

Place the trivet in the Pressure Pot and put the chicken strips on the trivet.

Cook the chicken using steam mode for 15 minutes.

Do a natural pressure release.

Meanwhile, place the lettuce and sliced tomato on the bread slices.

Add the cooked chicken strips to make the sandwiches.

Enjoy!

Nutrition:

Calories 212,

Fat 7.8,

Fiber 1,

Carbs 17.2,

Protein 17.9

Mediterranean Creamy Deviled Eggs

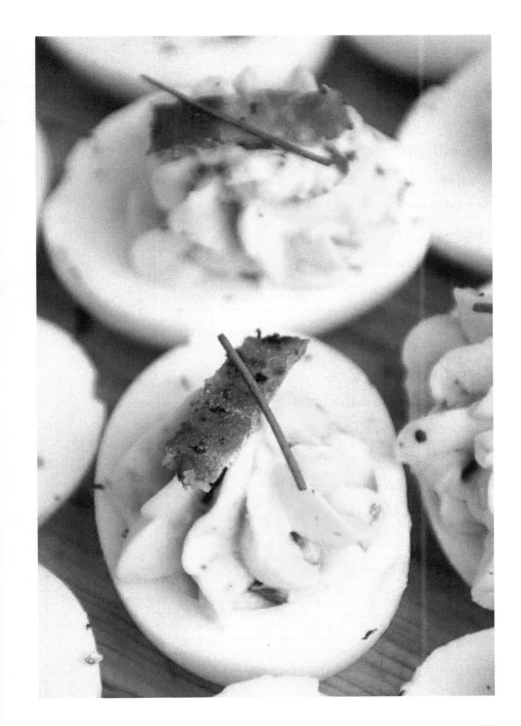

Difficulty Level: 2/5

Preparation Time: 10 minutes

Cooking time: 2 minutes

Servings: 4

Ingredients:

2 eggs

1 cup water

1 tablespoon cream

1 teaspoon mayo

½ teaspoon ground black pepper

1 teaspoon oregano

1 teaspoon cilantro

Directions:

Pour the water into the Pressure Pot.

Add the eggs and close the lid.

Cook the eggs on High pressure for 2 minutes.

Do a natural pressure release.

Cool the eggs in the ice water.

Peel the eggs.

Cut the eggs into halves and remove the egg yolks.

Put the egg yolks, mayo, ground black pepper, oregano, cilantro, and cream in a blender.

Blend the mixture well.

Fill the egg whites with the egg yolk mixture.

Enjoy!

Nutrition:

Calories 53,

Fat 4.2,

Fiber 0.2,

Carbs 1.2,

Protein 2.9

Fish Scones
Difficulty Level: 2/5

Preparation Time: 15 minutes

Cooking time: 10 minutes

Servings: 8

Ingredients:

8 oz. puff pastry

7 oz. tuna, canned

1 egg, whisked

1 teaspoon salt

1 teaspoon ground coriander

½ teaspoon ground black pepper

1 tablespoon olive oil

1 teaspoon dried dill

Directions:

Roll out the puff pastry.

Combine the whisked egg, canned tuna, salt, ground coriander, ground black pepper, and dried dill.

Stir the mixture well.

Cut the puff pastry into medium squares.

Place a small amount of the tuna mixture in each puff pastry square.

Secure the edges of the puff pastry in the shape of the scones.

Sprinkle the scones with the olive oil.

Place the scones in a baking pan and place the pan in the Pressure Pot bowl.

Cook the fish scones for 10 minutes on High pressure.

Do a natural pressure release.

Serve the cooked scones and enjoy!

Nutrition Value:

Calories 226,

Fat 15.1,

Fiber 0.5,

Carbs 13,

Protein 9.4

Green Beans with Yogurt Drizzle

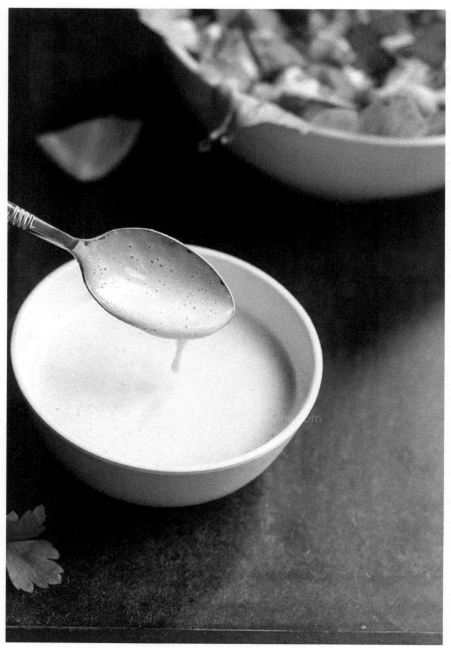

Difficulty Level: 2/5

Preparation time: 10 minutes

Cooking time: 5 minutes

Servings: 4

Ingredients:

1 pound of green beans (thin, trimmed)

3 tablespoons extra-virgin olive oil (divided)

1 red bell pepper (chopped)

1/2 cup Greek yogurt

1/4 cup grated Parmesan cheese

2 lemon juice teaspoons

1/2 teaspoon anchovy paste

1 clove garlic (chopped)

black olives (very small, for garnish)

fresh parsley (for garnish)

Directions:

Steam or cook green beans in boiling water to desired softness. Drain. Heat 1 tablespoon oil in a skillet and cook 10-inch pepper over medium heat, stirring occasionally for 4 minutes or until softened.

Add green beans and toss to coat. Combine remaining ingredients except olives in a microwave-safe bowl and cook at HIGH temp. for 30 seconds, stirring once, until warm.

Arrange green beans on a serving platter. Top with red peppers and olives. Serve sauce over vegetables. Garnish with fresh parsley leaves.

Nutrition: (Per serving)

190 Calories;

0.14g fat;

0.12g carbs;

0.6g protein;

Roast Vegetables with Tomatoes, Feta and Basil

Difficulty Level: 2/5

Preparation time: 15 minutes

Cooking time: 15 minutes

Servings: 4

Ingredients:

zucchini (thinly sliced, about 200 g)

olive oil

salt

pepper

2 cloves

eggplant (cut into small cubes, approximately 200 g)

bell pepper (medium size, color of your choice, cut into small cubes, 1)

cherry tomatoes (cut in half, 8)

feta cheese (broken into pieces, approximately 100 g / 3 1/2 oz)

10 fresh basil leaves

Directions:

Heat a slash or olive oil in a large pan and sauté the zucchini on medium-high heat until golden brown with a little bite. Season with salt and pepper to taste, transfer to a plate and set aside.

Put the pan back on the heat, pour in a splash of olive oil, stir in the garlic and let it turn golden (not brown!) For about 1 minute. Add the eggplant and bell pepper, season with salt and pepper and sauté until golden and soft. Take the pan off the heat, mix in the zucchini and tomatoes and season to taste. Stir in the feta and basil and serve immediately, or as a warm salad, with fresh ciabatta bread.

Nutrition: (Per serving)

90 Calories;

0.7g fat;

0.6g carbs;

0.2g protein;

Roasted Broccoli & Tomatoes
Difficulty Level: 2/5

Preparation time: 5 minutes

Cooking time: 20 minutes

Servings: 4

Ingredients:

12 ounces of broccoli (crowns, trimmed and cut into bite-size florets, about 4 cups)

1 cup grape tomatoes

1 tablespoon extra-virgin olive oil

2 cloves of garlic

1/4 teaspoon salt

1/2 teaspoon grated lemon zest (freshly)

1 tablespoon lemon juice

10 pitted black olives (sliced)

1 teaspoon of dried oregano

2 teaspoons capers (rinsed, optional)

Directions:

Preheat oven to 450 ° F.

Throw broccoli, tomatoes, oil, garlic and salt in a large bowl until evenly covered. Spread in an even layer on a baking sheet. Bake until the broccoli starts to brown, 10 to 13 minutes.

Meanwhile, mix lemon zest and juice, olives, oregano and capers (if used) in a large bowl. Add the roasted vegetables; stir to combine. Serve hot.

Nutrition: (Per serving)

70 Calories;

0.35g fat;

0.9g carbs;

0.3g protein

Grilled Zucchini with Tomato and Feta
Difficulty Level: 2/5

Preparation time: 5 minutes

Cooking time: 12 minutes

Servings: 6

Ingredients:

3 zucchini (or zucchini and yellow squash, tops removed, cut in half lengthwise)

freshly ground pepper (bars)

1/2 teaspoon of garlic powder

extra virgin olive oil

1/2 lemon (about 1 tbsp lemon juice)

1 whole lemon

1/2 cup of crumbled feta cheese

3 pearl tomatoes (chopped, drained in a colander)

1 green onion (both white and green, finely chopped)

Directions:

If cooking on gas grill, lightly oil the grate and preheat grill to medium-low. (OR, heat and cast iron skillet or indoor griddle over medium heat.)

Brush zucchini generously with extra virgin olive oil on both sides. Season zucchini (particularly flesh side) with salt, freshly ground pepper, and oregano

Place zucchini, flesh-side down, on the preheated grill (or indoor griddle). Grill for 3 to 5 minutes until soft and nicely charred, then turn on back side and grill for another 3 to 5 minutes until this side is also tender and gains some color. (If using an indoor skillet or griddle, you may need to adjust heat to medium-high.)

Remove zucchini from heat and let's cool enough to handle.

To create zucchini boats, use a small spoon to scoop out the flesh into a small bowl (do not discard.) Squeeze all liquid out of zucchini flesh (you might use a linen kitchen towel or paper towel to do this.)

Now add zucchini flesh to a mixing bowl. Add the remaining ingredients (cherry tomatoes, green onions, feta, mint, parsley, lemon zest, and small splash or lemon juice). Sprinkle a little more oregano, if you like, and add a drizzle or extra virgin olive oil. Mix everything together to make the filling.

Spoon the filling mixture into the prepared zucchini boats and arrange on a serving platter. Enjoy!

Nutrition: (Per serving)

90 Calories;

0.6g fat;

0.7g carbs;

0.3g protein;

0mg of cholesterol;

150mg sodium

Taziki's Mediterranean Cafés Basmati Rice
Difficulty Level: 2/5

Preparation time: 10 minutes

Cooking time: 20 minutes

Servings: 4

Ingredients:

2 cups basmati rice (long grain Indian Basmati rice)

3 cups of water

4 ounces of unsalted butter (melted)

1 teaspoon of salt

1 teaspoon pepper

4 lemon juice (lemons)

1/2 cup parsley (fresh chopped)

Directions:

Put water and rice in an 8-liter pan with a lid.

Bring the rice to the boil quickly while it is covered.

When the water boils, set the temperature low.

Bake for 12 to 15 minutes until the rice is fluffy.

Remove the pan from the burner and let the rice stand for 2 to 5 minutes.

Pour cooked rice into a medium-sized mixing bowl.

Add melted butter, salt, pepper, lemon juice and parsley.

Stir until it has cooled completely.

Nutrition: (Per serving)

560 Calories;

0.24g fat;

0.79g carbs;

0.7g protein

Roasted Broccoli & Tomatoes
Difficulty Level: 2/5

Preparation time: 5 minutes

Cooking time: 20 minutes

Servings: 4

Ingredients:

12 ounces of broccoli (crowns, trimmed and cut into bite-size florets, about 4 cups)

1 cup grape tomatoes

1 tablespoon extra-virgin olive oil

2 cloves of garlic (minced)

1/4 teaspoon salt

1/2 teaspoon grated lemon zest (freshly)

1 tablespoon lemon juice

10 pitted black olives (sliced)

1 teaspoon of dried oregano

2 teaspoons capers (rinsed, optional)

Directions:

Preheat oven to 450 ° F. Toss broccoli, tomatoes, oil, garlic and salt in a large bowl until evenly coated. Spread in an even layer on a baking sheet. Bake until the broccoli starts to brown, 10 to 13 minutes.

Meanwhile, combine lemon zest and juice, olives, oregano and capers (if using) in a large bowl. Add the roasted vegetables; stir to combine. Serve hot.

Nutrition: (Per serving)

70 Calories;

0.35g fat;

0.9g carbs;

0.3g protein;

Green Beans Mediterranean Style

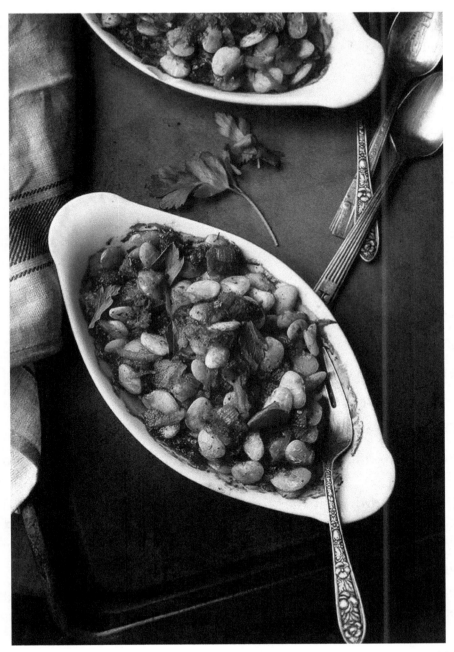

Difficulty Level: 2/5

Preparation time: 5 minutes

Cooking time: 10 minutes

Servings: 6

Ingredients:

12 ounces of haricot verts (Fresh, French Green Beans, See Note 1)

1 1/2 cups cherry tomatoes

1/3 cup pitted kalamata olives (Small)

2 cups bread cubes (1/2 ", See Note 2)

1/2 oregano teaspoon

1/2 teaspoon of salt

4 tablespoons extra virgin olive oil (divided)

1/4 teaspoon Dijon mustard

1 tablespoon balsamic vinegar (White)

1 ounce of feta cheese

1 pinch red pepper flake

Directions:

Preheat oven to 375 ºF (Conventional), or 350 ºF for Convection (fan).

In a large bowl, place the green beans, tomatoes, olives and bread cubes. Drizzle with 3 T olive oil, the oregano, and 1/2 t salt. Mix until all pieces are coated.

Spread onto large Sheet Pan.

Place in oven for 15-20 minutes, until croutons are crispy, and beans are tender. In my oven, this took about 18 minutes

Make the dressing. In a small container with a member, mix the Dijon mustard, balsamic vinegar and the remaining tablespoon of olive oil. Add a pinch of salt and a few changes to freshly ground pepper. Sprinkle with the green beans. Place in a serving dish.

Crumble and sprinkle the feta cheese and a pinch of red pepper flake (if desired) over the top and serve while it is hot.

Nutrition: (Per serving)

160 Calories;

0.11g fat;

0.13g carbs;

0.3g protein;

Italian-style Broccoli
Difficulty Level: 2/5

Preparation time: 5 minutes

Cooking time: 25 minutes

Servings: 4

Ingredients:

3 cloves of garlic (diced)

1/2 yellow onion (diced)

3 tablespoons olive oil

1 pound broccoli florets (steamed, fresh or frozen)

1/4 cup black olives (finely chopped)

3/4 teaspoon of salt

Directions:

About medium heat, sauté the onion and garlic in the oil for 2-3 minutes until the onions start to turn color.

Add in the broccoli and lower the heat. Toss the pan to make sure the broccoli soaks up the oil.

Also add in the olives and distribute throughout the dish. Serve hot.

Nutrition: (Per serving)

150 Calories;

0.11g fat;

0.10g carbs;

0.4g protein;

Zucchini Mediterranean
Difficulty Level: 2/5

Preparation time: 5 minutes

Cooking time: 25 minutes

Servings: 4

Ingredients:

4 zucchini

2 tablespoons olive oil

2 tablespoons of vinegar

1 garlic (mashed)

1/2 teaspoon basil

1/2 oregano teaspoon

salt (to taste)

pepper (to taste)

Directions:

Wash, trim, and slice zucchini

Saute in oil until slightly soft.

Drizzle vinegar about zucchini while cooking.

Add garlic, basil, oregano, salt, and pepper.

Toss to coat well.

Serve hot or cold.

Nutrition: (Per serving)

100 Calories;

0.7g fat;

0.8g carbs;

0.2g protein

Greek Couscous
Difficulty Level: 2/5

Preparation time: 5 minutes

Cooking time: 20 minutes

Servings: 4

Ingredients:

1 cup of couscous

1 cup of water

2/3 cup peppers (diced, sweet, bell ... whatever suits your fancy)

1/2 cup sun-dried tomatoes (diced)

2/3 cup kalamata olives (chopped)

3 tablespoons juices (oils from tomatoes and olives)

4 ounces of crumbled feta cheese

parsley (generous sprinkle or, I used dried, but you can use fresh if you have it)

Directions:

Prepare couscous as indicated on the package. (Mine says to boil the water, add couscous, stir quickly and remove from the heat; let stand for 5 minutes). I have skipped both butter and salt.

Mix the peppers, tomatoes and olives well in a large bowl.

Add couscous and stir, breaking up the large pieces.

Add the juices and / or oils from the tomatoes and olive to the couscous as needed to keep dish moist, but not wet. Couscous will absorb liquid quickly, so be generous and work fast.

Once the couscous and vegetables are mixed well, add feta and stir to combine.

Sprinkle parsley just before serving. Enjoy!

Nutrition: (Per serving)

330 Calories;

0.1g fat;

0.52g carbs;

0.13g protein;

Mushroom Couscous

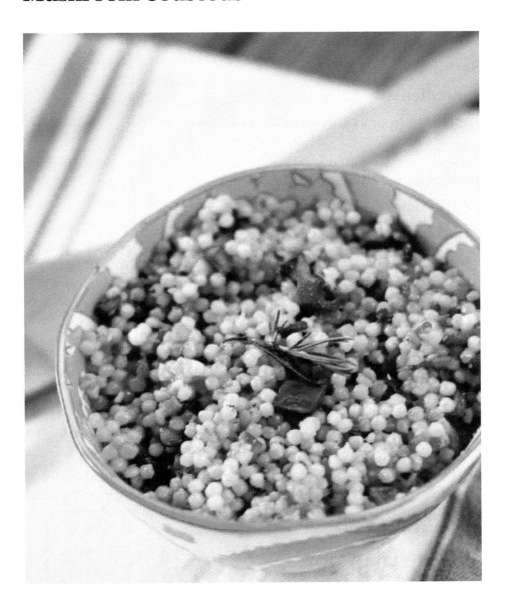

Difficulty Level: 2/5

Preparation time: 5 minutes

Cooking time: 30 minutes

Servings: 4

Ingredients:

1/2 cup couscous (uncooked)

1 cup of water

1 tablespoon butter

7 mushrooms (sliced)

2 carrots (sliced & cooked)

2 tablespoons chive (chopped)

1 teaspoon garlic powder

1 1/2 herb teaspoons (Italian, blend)

1 tablespoon lemon juice

salt / pepper

Directions:

Add couscous and water in a medium saucepan. Bake for 5 - 10 minutes over medium heat until the couscous is cooked.

Melt butter in a frying pan. Add sliced mushrooms and cook for 5 minutes. Add carrots, cooked couscous, chopped chives, garlic powder, Italian spice mix and lemon juice. Bake for about 5 - 10 minutes. Season with salt and pepper.

Nutrition: (Per serving)

150 Calories;

0.35g fat;

0.25g carbs;

0.5g protein

Lightning Source UK Ltd.
Milton Keynes UK
UKHW020644010621
384724UK00004B/38